Fertility Matters™

A Natural Women's Fertility Monitoring System

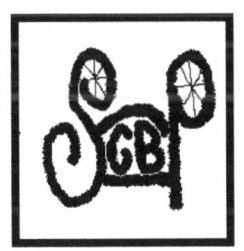

St. Croix Birth & Parenting
Stillwater, Minnesota

Additional copies of this workbook can be ordered from:

St. Croix Birth & Parenting
15072 62nd Street North #2
Oak Park Heights, MN 55082
www.stcroixbirth.com

Fertility Matters

Table of Contents

The Fertility Matters™ Method...

- Is a simple, highly effective Sympto-Thermal Method of Natural Family Planning, for those times during your childbearing years when you discern a need to postpone pregnancy
- Provides fertility counseling services throughout your entire childbearing years
- Encourages you to take good care of yourself to preserve your fertility, something that is important for your long-term health and well-being, as well as that of your children
- Provides a helpful snapshot of your gynecological health from cycle to cycle, giving you and your personal fertility advisor important information you can use to enhance your fertility using natural means
- Helps hone habits you can use to grow in holiness, and helps you and your spouse to build a strong marriage, joyful family, and solid financial foundation
- Is rooted in Catholic teachings on marriage and family
- Includes perspectives and ideas from many Christian leaders and scholars

The Fertility Matters Method

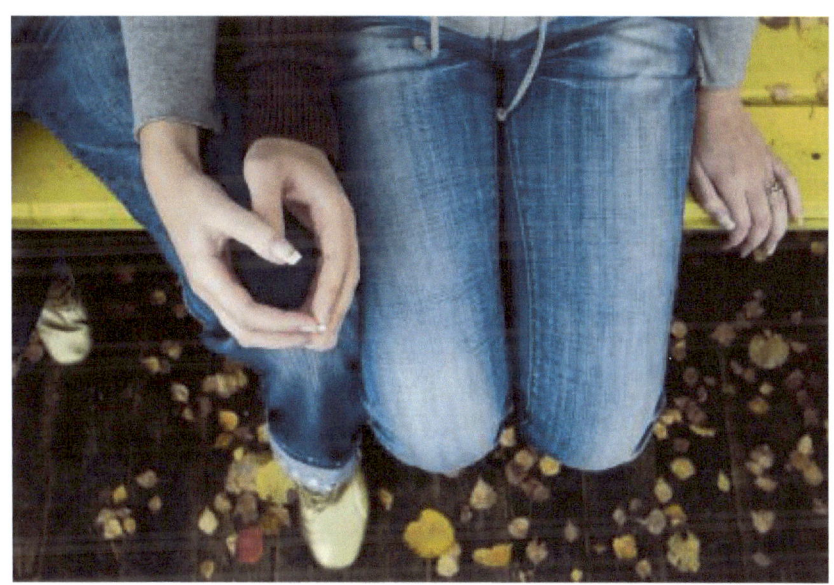

Fertility naturally springs from a healthy body.
Healthy babies come from healthy parents.
~Christelle J. K. Hagen, CCE, FE

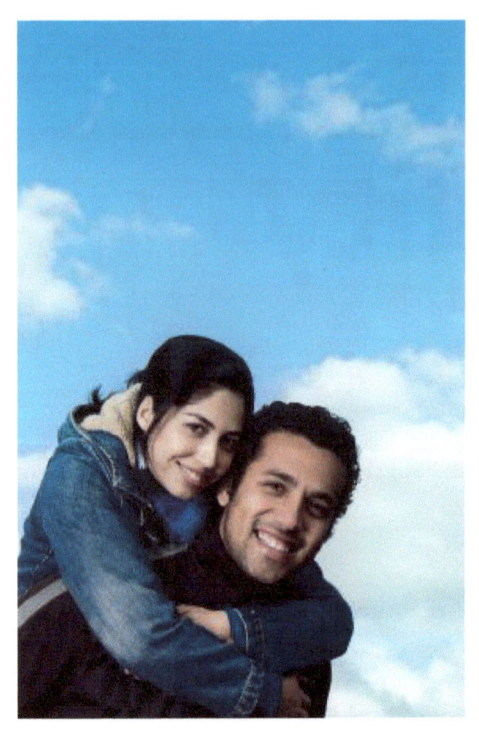

The Fertility Matters™ Method for Natural Family Planning

The Fertility Matters™ Method is a "Sympto-Thermal" Method of Natural Family Planning (NFP).

o **Know your fertility status on a daily basis**: know if she is very unlikely, may possibly, or is highly likely to become pregnant.

o **Is completely natural**: uses no drugs or devices, except for a thermometer! There are no side effects and no risks.

o **Works! Highly effective**: 99% effective at preventing pregnancy when used correctly.

o **Is simple to use**, once you know how to observe and interpret your signs of fertility. We keep things simple for you and expect a lot from our educators and counselors. Instead of teaching you many complicated rules, we teach one basic rule. If you are ever in a situation where you do not know how to apply the basic rules, simply contact your fertility advisor who knows many rules and can help you determine when you are no longer fertile.

o **Helps strengthen your marriage**: Our Nurturing the GIFTs of Life & Love goal-setting process helps prevent "NFP drop-outs" *and* stress on your marriage by giving you practical tips on how to continue to practice romance and build your marriage while using NFP.

 ## What does 'Sympto-Thermal' mean?

- "Sympto" means signs or symptoms
- "Thermal" means temperature

- A "**Sympto-Thermal**" method of NFP is one in which a woman learns how to check her natural signs or symptoms of fertility as well as take her temperature daily. By learning how to interpret the changes in her symptoms and temperature, you can tell if she is fertile or not.

The Fertility Matters™ Method for Natural Fertility Support

The Fertility Matters™ Method gives you access to confidential, private fertility counseling appointments, *from your initial program through menopause!*

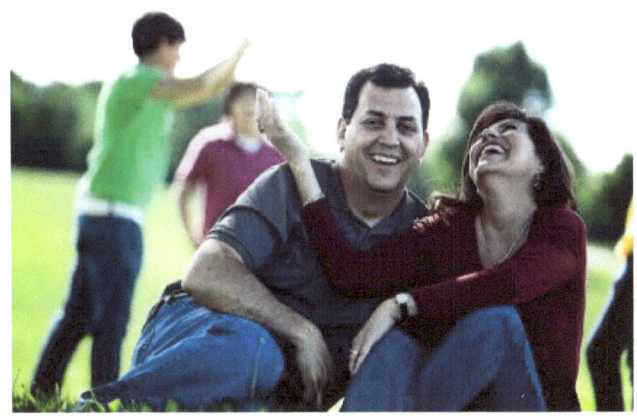

- **Helps gauge and strengthen your fertility**: using the information you gather about your signs of fertility, your fertility counselor can assess your gynecological health and suggest improvements that help support or may enhance your fertility. In the future, we are planning to expand our fertility counseling services by launching a Certified Fertility Midwife (CFM) certification program. A CFM will be a highly trained health care practitioner who will be a certified Natural Family Planning educator and counselor, and a Professional Herbalist. A Certified Fertility Midwife will be fully qualified to help enhance fertility using a variety of natural (non-surgical, non-pharmacological) healing modalities.
- **Helps build your health**: natural fertility support is achieved by common-sense health practices with proven effectiveness, such as reducing your stress, getting adequate rest, eating well, exercising moderately, and maintaining a healthy body balance. Even if you are not planning a pregnancy in the near future, maintaining normal fertility is important for your general health and well-being.
- **Provides pre-conceptual care**: Our programs are excellent for helping you to prepare for conception.
- **May detect unknown health problems**: Many couples assume that they have normal fertility, when in actuality they do not. This method can provide a warning that you may have a medical problem, allowing early intervention.
- **Provides referrals to qualified health care providers**: Our fertility counselors are trained to refer you to qualified NFP-only medical doctors or other health care providers, if necessary.

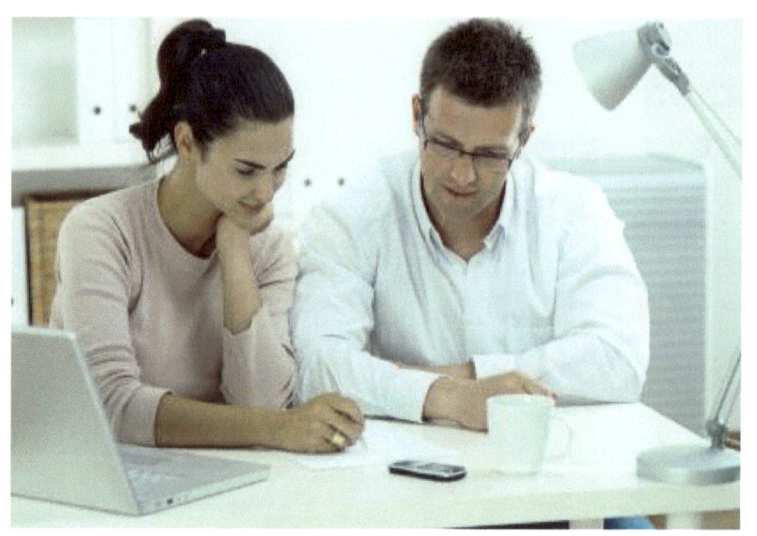

The Fertility Matters™ Method for *real* "Family Planning"

- **Makes each moment a gift:** A crucial part of the Fertility Matters™ Method is our exclusive "Nurturing the GIFTs of Life & Love" goal-setting process. By systematically setting and achieving goals in up to six major areas of your life, you will be amazed at the increased peace and joy you will experience in your daily life.
- **Puts First Things First**: by planning how you will spend your day, and prioritizing what you are planning to do, you can plan to do the most important things: prayer, care of yourself, and time with your spouse and your children.
- **Helps you grow in self-giving love**: by planning ways to effectively express your love for others, you will become a more effective giver (even when you don't feel like it)!
- **Leads to life-changing decisions**: While we usually think of "family planning" as something that helps a woman to avoid becoming pregnant, "Family Planning" in our classes means something very different—planning your personal and family goals and taking steps toward achieving them. Couples find that decisions about family size that may have been made based on emotions alone or less important reasons may change once you know the direction you want your family to go.
- **Is an essential component of natural fertility support & enhancement**: While the GIFTs goal-setting process might seem unrelated to fertility education, it is actually an essential component of supporting or enhancing your fertility, because the goal-setting process is the "method" by which you will incorporate the changes necessary for fertility support or enhancement.

The Fertility Matters™ Method: a method for all Christians

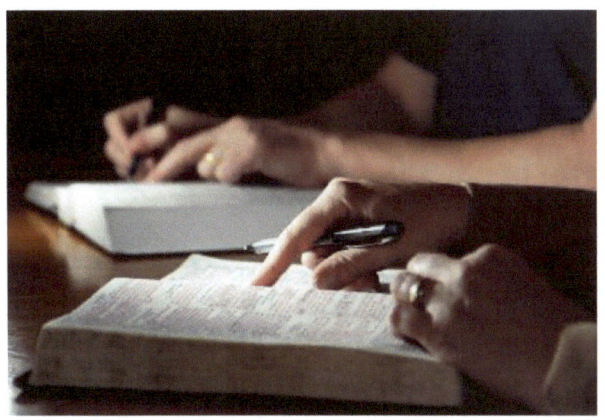

- The Fertility Matters™ Method is a **method of Natural Family Planning with roots in Catholic teachings on marriage & family.**
  - Each class session includes valuable teachings about human sexuality, marriage, and family life. We would be happy to point you to the original documents, in case you wish to read them on their own.
  - In areas where Christian bodies disagree, we present Catholic teaching, because we believe that it clearly articulates Biblical teachings on marriage, the blessing of children, and the virtue of prudence; and also protects children, marriages, and families.

- The Fertility Matters™ Method is **for all Christians.**
  - We strive to make every session equally welcoming for all Christians. Therefore, we ask program participants to limit discussions of theological and other differences among Christians to outside-of-class times.
  - Each session includes Bible passages for discussion and study.
  - Quotations from Catholic, Protestant and other Christian leaders and scholars are included.

Today, however, there is a resurgence among young evangelical Protestant couples who seek to recapture a holy vision of marriage that is not possible with contraception. They are excitedly embracing the integrated view of human worth, sexuality, and reproduction held by key Protestant Reformers such as Luther, Calvin and Wesley—a view that human life carries a spark of divine life, not just in the spiritual realm, but in the physical and biological realm as well... Consequently, growing numbers of couples are embracing Natural Family Planning (NFP) as the way to naturally and faithfully build Christian families.

~ *Cindy Omlin, "Building Holy Families the Natural Way"*
"Leadership U" website (leaderu.com);
Christian Leadership Ministries—Campus Crusade for Christ, International

Fertility Matters™ Method Educators & Counselors:

- Understand the importance of fertility
- Want to help you support or enhance your fertility and strengthen all areas of your life

All fertility educators and counselors affiliated with the Fertility Matters Method agree with the following statements:

- Children are the natural fruit of marriage. Any device, procedure or practice that frustrates the natural life-giving potential of the marital embrace or destroys its fruit is unethical.

- Natural family planning methods may be utilized by couples wishing to postpone pregnancy for just reasons, because such methods preserve the life-giving potential of the marital embrace and its fruit.

- Natural conception is best for couples and their babies. All aids to conception which assist the couple to achieve natural conception within the context of the marital embrace are licit. Any practice or procedure that attempts to create a new human life outside of the context of the marital embrace is unethical.

- Many couples who struggle with infertility or repeat miscarriages can achieve healthy pregnancies if they practice fertility awareness, along with changes in lifestyle such as: a healthier diet, moderate exercise, stress reduction, and natural hormone balancing. Referrals to NFP-only physicians will be made, whenever appropriate.

Fertility Matters

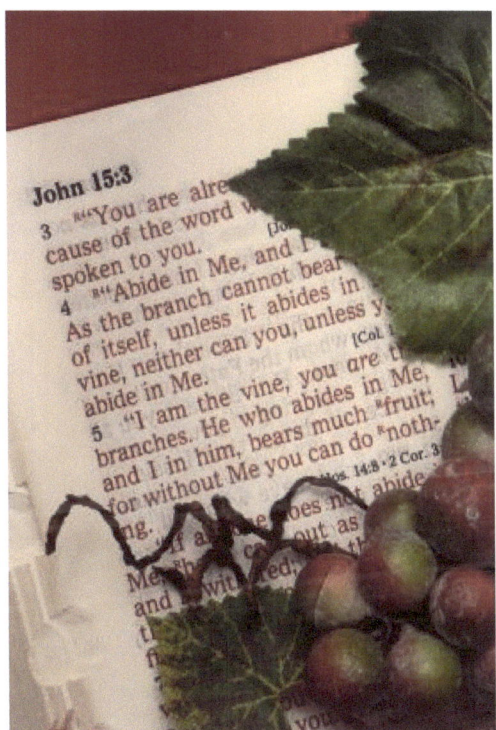

Your wife will be like a fruitful vine within your house...
Thus is the man blessed who fears the LORD.
~Psalm 128:3, 4

Up for Discussion

Why Fertility Matters

Why do *you* think fertility matters? Discuss with your fiancé(e), spouse or another class participant and write down your answers here. During your instructor's speech or class discussion, feel free to add new ideas to this list.

God's Marvelous Designs for Man & Woman

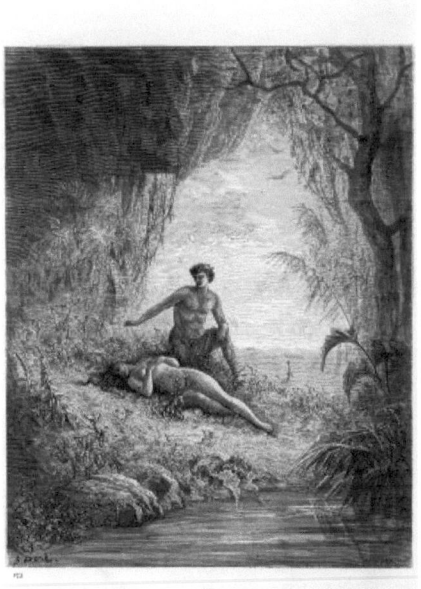

So the LORD God cast a deep sleep on the man, and while he was asleep, he took out one of his ribs and closed up its place with flesh. The LORD God then built up into a woman the rib that he had taken from the man. When he brought her to the man, the man said: 'This one, at last, is bone of my bones and flesh of my flesh; This one shall be called 'woman,' for out of 'her man' this one has been taken.
~Gen. 2:21-23 NAB

How God Made Men: **Male Anatomy & Physiology**

Once the class and your fertility educator agree that all the labels are in the right places, record the names of these parts of a man's body.

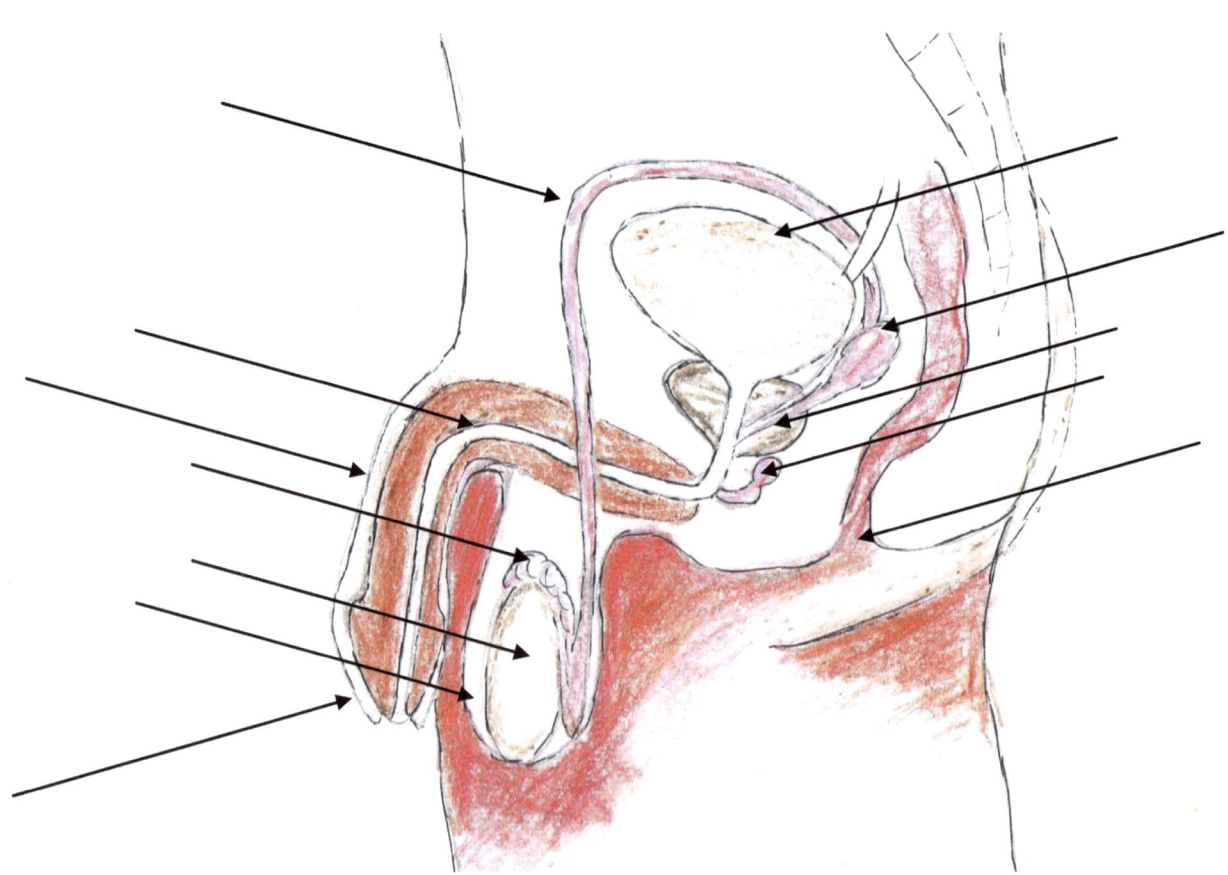

How God Made Women: **Female Anatomy**

Once the class and your fertility educator agree that all the labels are in the right places, record the names of these parts of a woman's body.

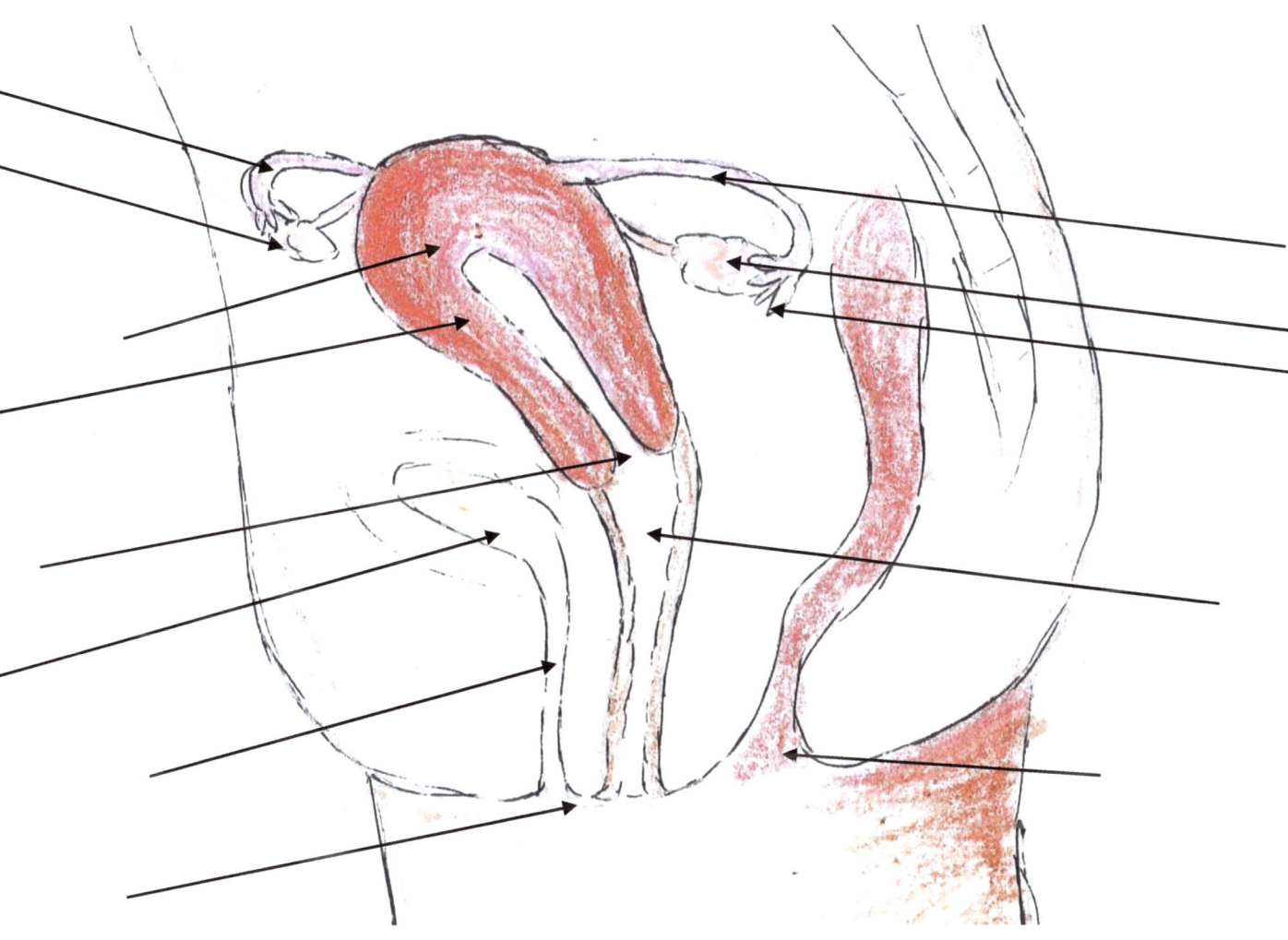

How God Made Women: **Your Fertility Cycle**

Draw the correct phase of the moon in the boxes above each part of a woman's fertility cycle, matching the full moon phase with the woman's time of maximum fertility.

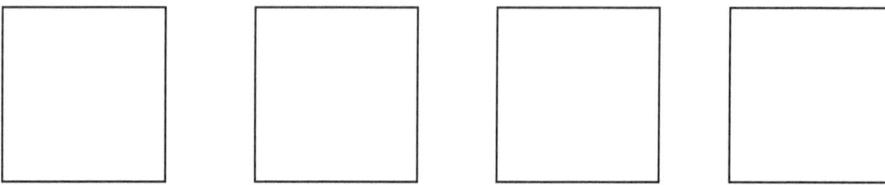

Menses + Dry Days   Fluid Begins   Ovulation   Fluid Dries Up

Important! The analogy of the phases of the moon is intended to help you remember the normal waxing and waning of a woman's fertility throughout each cycle. It doesn't mean that a woman's phases of fertility will necessarily match up with the true phases of the moon.

A Typical Fertility Cycle

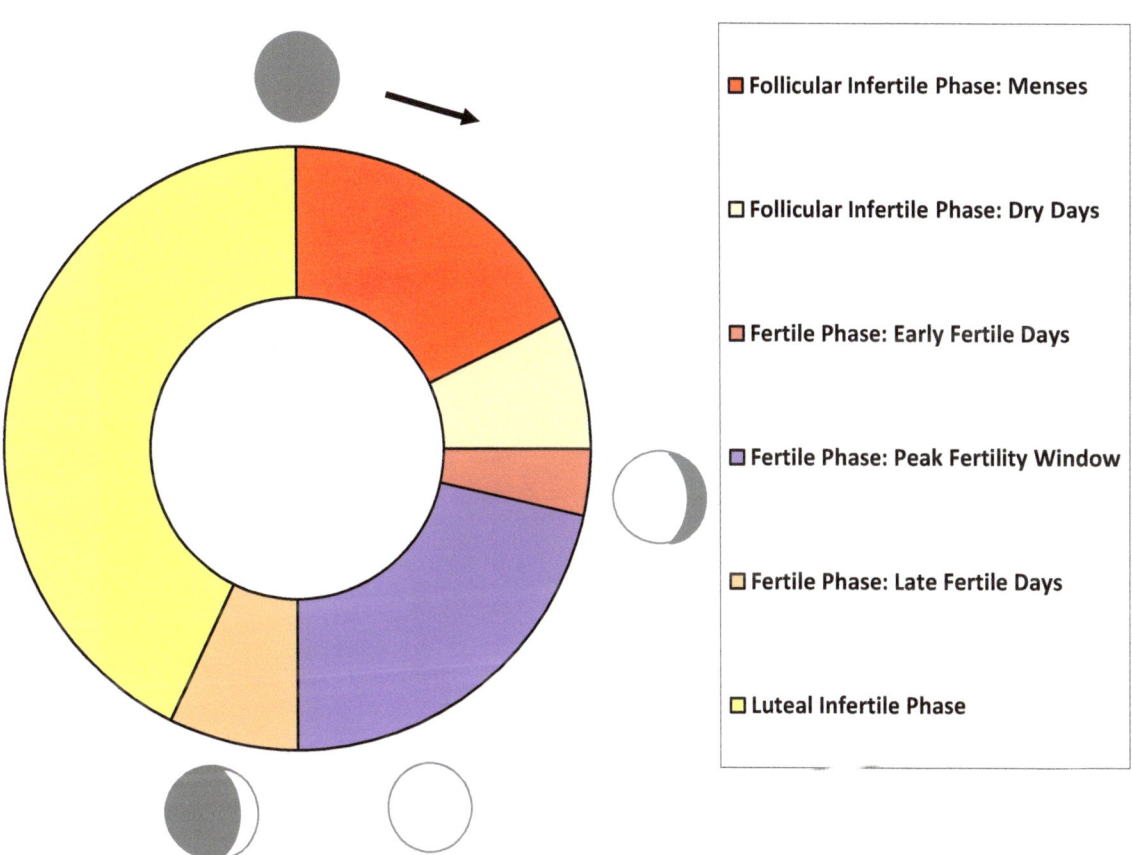

- Follicular Infertile Phase: Menses
- Follicular Infertile Phase: Dry Days
- Fertile Phase: Early Fertile Days
- Fertile Phase: Peak Fertility Window
- Fertile Phase: Late Fertile Days
- Luteal Infertile Phase

Your Fertility Cycle

As your fertility educator describes the phases of a woman's fertility cycle, write the answers on the appropriate spaces on this table. Your instructor will go over the correct answers, so you can change them if you make a mistake.

Name & length of this phase of cycle				
Hormones for this part of the cycle				
Changes in her ovaries				
Changes in her uterus				
Changes in her cervix				
Changes in basal body temperature				
Likelihood of pregnancy				

Your Fertility Cycle: **The Follicular Infertile Phase**

Write down these facts about this phase of a woman's fertility cycle.

Nickname:

First Day of the Follicular Infertile Phase:

How you can tell you are in this phase:

Hormones dominant during this phase:

How do hormones affect a woman's ovaries during this phase?

How do hormones affect a woman's uterus during this phase?

How do hormones affect a woman's cervix during this phase?

How do hormones affect a woman's temperature during this phase?

What is the likelihood of pregnancy during this phase?

Anything else you should remember about this phase?

Last Day of the Follicular Infertile Phase:

The Follicular Infertile Phase

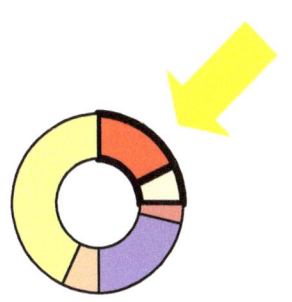

If you are using detailed charting, remember to make note of the following aspects of your menstrual bleeding:

1. Length of your period
2. Quantity
3. Color
4. Consistency
5. Symptoms

Your Fertile Phase: **The Early Fertile Days**

Write down these facts about this part of a woman's fertility cycle.

First Day of the Early Fertile Days:

How you can tell you are in the Early Fertile Days:

Hormones dominant:

How do hormones affect a woman's ovaries during this time?

How do hormones affect a woman's uterus during this time?

How do hormones affect a woman's cervix during this time?

How do hormones affect a woman's temperature during this time?

What is the likelihood of pregnancy?

Anything else you should remember?

Last Day of the Early Fertile Days:

The Fertile Phase: Early Fertile Days

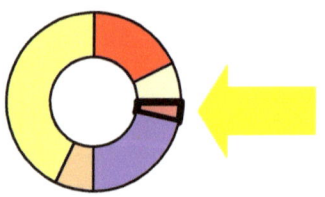

Typical
FAST Check observations
during the Early Fertile Days:

F=Feel...a bit slippery
A=Amount...a little
S=See...shimmering or shininess
T=Touch test...no stretch, or very little stretch
(less than ¾ inch or 2 cm)

Your Fertile Phase: **Peak Fertility Window**

Write down these facts about this part of a woman's fertility cycle.

First Day of the Peak Fertility Window:

How you can tell you are in the Peak Fertility Window:

Hormones dominant:

How do hormones affect a woman's ovaries during this time?

How do hormones affect a woman's uterus during this time?

How do hormones affect a woman's cervix during this time?

How do hormones affect a woman's body temperature during this time?

What is the likelihood of pregnancy?

Anything else you should remember?

Last Day of the Peak Fertility Window:

The Fertile Phase: Peak Fertility Window

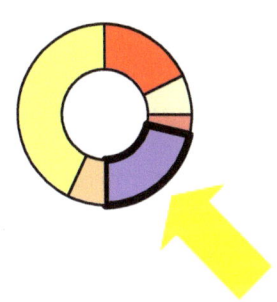

Typical FAST Check observations during the Peak Fertility Window:

F=Feel...very slippery
A=Amount...lots
S=See...clear stretchy fluid, like raw egg white
T=Touch test...stretchy (more than ¾ inch or 2 cm)

Your Fertile Phase: **Other Signs ovulation is near**

Fill in the blanks as you listen to your fertility educator.

Other biological signs you can observe or become aware of that indicate fertility are:

1. Changes in a woman's _____, specifically, when she is most fertile it is:
    a. open or closed?
    b. high or low?
    c. firm or soft?

2. Pain occurring near the area of the woman's _____, called: _____

3. Some women, especially those who have given birth before, may notice jabbing pains inside their _____ when they are near to ovulation.

4. It is common for a woman's libido to _____ around the time of ovulation.

5. Occasionally, a woman may notice some _____ near the time of ovulation.

6. Lastly, you may also notice changes in your _____ around the time of ovulation; for example, teariness, depression, anxiety or anger.

Ovulation Testing Products

Need more help determining if you are fertile? Consider purchasing an ovulation testing product. Your fertility educator will discuss several options. If you need help choosing, ask your fertility advisor about the various options during your next fertility counseling appointment.

Your Fertile Phase: **Late Fertile Days**

Write down these facts about this part of a woman's fertility cycle.

First Day of the Late Fertile Days:

How you can tell you are in the Late Fertile Days:

Hormones dominant:

How do hormones affect a woman's ovaries during this time?

How do hormones affect a woman's uterus during this time?

How do hormones affect a woman's cervix during this time?

How do hormones affect a woman's body temperature during this time?

What is the likelihood of pregnancy?

Anything else you should remember?

Last Day of the Late Fertile Days:

**The Fertile Phase:
Late Fertile Days**

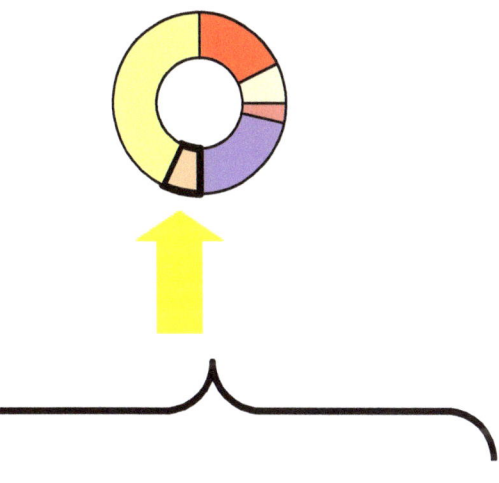

*Typical
FAST Check observations
during the Late Fertile Days:*

F=Feel…a little slippery or dry
A=Amount…not much or none
S=See…shimmery or shiny cervical fluid
T=Touch test…not stretchy (less than ¾ inch or 2 cm)

Your Fertility Cycle: **The Luteal Infertile Phase**

Write down these facts about this phase of a woman's fertility cycle.

The Luteal Infertile Phase

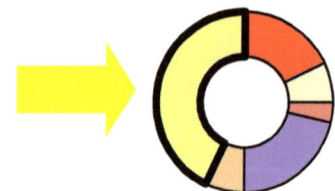

Nickname for this Phase:

First Day of the Luteal Infertile Phase:

How you can tell you are in the Luteal Infertile Phase:

Hormones dominant:

How do hormones affect a woman's ovaries during this phase?

How do hormones affect a woman's uterus during this phase?

How do hormones affect a woman's cervix during this phase?

How do hormones affect a woman's body temperature during this phase?

What is the likelihood of pregnancy?

Anything else you should remember?

Last Day of the Luteal Infertile Phase:

Typical FAST Check observations during the Luteal Infertile Phase:

F=Feel...dry
A=Amount...none
S=See...nothing
T=Touch test...nothing to test

Late in your cycle you may notice some cervical fluid, but it is not related to fertility.

20

Charting Your Signs of Fertility

The following table contains observations "Nikki" made in her second cycle of charting. Using the practice chart and the symbol sheet in your Chart Booklet, record Nikki's observations on the practice chart.

Cycle Day	Temperature	Bleeding & Cervical Fluid Observations
1	98.1	Moderate menstrual bleeding
2	98.2	Moderate menstrual bleeding
3	98.0	Moderate menstrual bleeding
4	98.3	Moderate menstrual bleeding
5	97.8	Light menstrual bleeding
6	97.9	Spotting
7	97.7	Dry
8	97.9	Dry
9	97.8	Dry
10	97.9	Sticky
11	98.0	Sticky
12	98.2	Wet feelings, Stretchy cervical fluid, Yellowish color, Lots
13	98.0	Stretchy cervical fluid, Clear color, Less
14	97.8	Stretchy cervical fluid, Clear color, Less
15		Stretchy cervical fluid
16	98.4	Sticky
17	98.5	Sticky
18		Dry
19	98.5	Dry
20		Dry
21	98.5	Dry
22	98.1	Dry
23	98.4	
24	98.4	
25	98.6	
26	98.6	
27	98.6	
28	98.6	
29	98.4	
30	98.2	

Interpreting Your Signs of Fertility:
The Traffic Light Rule

By following these steps, you can determine when the Luteal Infertile Phase begins during a fertility cycle.

1. Mark the Pregnancy Intention on the chart.
   a. TTC=trying to conceive
   b. Open=open to a baby, but not actively trying to become pregnant
   c. TTA=trying to avoid or postpone pregnancy
   d. N/A=not applicable (for example, for single women using the method to improve women's health)
2. Be alert for a change from More-Fertile to Less-Fertile Cervical Fluid *that is associated with a rise in temperature.*
3. Correctly identify and mark "Peak Day" on your chart.
   a. Remember: Peak Day is the last day you observe More-Fertile Cervical Fluid during a fertility cycle. It is normally associated with a rise in your temperature.
   b. You will have more than one peak day if you have more than one patch of More-Fertile Cervical Fluid.
   c. Use a small "p" for any peak day that is not associated with a rise in your temperature. Use a capital "P" for the true Peak Day, the one that is associated with a rise in temperature (3 days of rising temps).
4. Draw a box around the Peak Fertility Window (PFW), in the Inter+Pk Fert row of the chart.
   a. The first day of the PFW is the first day of the cycle when you observe More-Fertile Cervical Fluid.
   b. The last day of the PFW is the day after a peak day (Peak Day+1).
   c. You will have several Peak Fertility Windows if you have more than 1 patch of More-Fertile Cervical Fluid.
5. Mark the first 4 dry or drying up days following Peak Day: red, red, yellow, green.
6. Draw a horizontal coverline across your chart.
   a. The coverline should be drawn 1/10[tho] F above the follicular phase temperatures that come *after* menstruation and *before* the first 3 elevated temperatures. The line may extend to the end of the chart.
   b. If you have one or two follicular phase temperatures that are very high compared to the others, you can ignore them.
7. Circle the first three temperatures after Peak Day that are above the coverline: red, yellow, green.
8. Locate the cycle day that has a "green light" from both the temperature and cervical fluid rows, *whichever comes last.* This is the first day of the Luteal Infertile Phase!
9. Draw a vertical LIP line down your chart between the last day of the Fertile Phase and the first day of the LIP.
   a. Your Luteal Infertile Phase begins on the evening of that cycle day.

According to the <u>Traffic Light Rule</u>:
You have reached the Luteal Infertile Phase
on the <u>evening</u> of the cycle day
that meets these conditions:

Since the last day you observed More-Fertile Cervical Fluid,
- ○ **at least four days have passed, AND**
- ○ **three of your temperatures have been <u>above</u> the coverline**

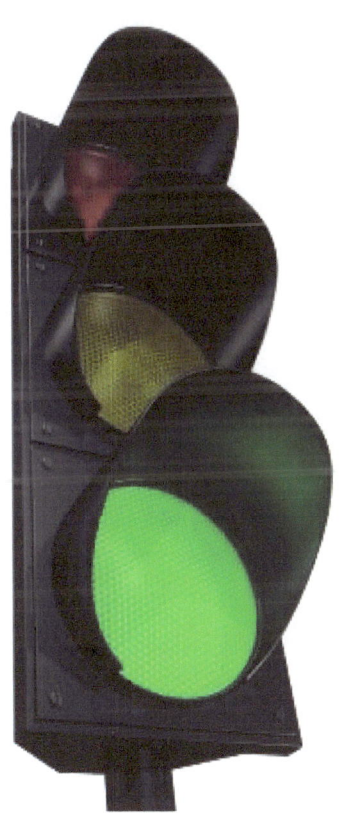

The Long Red Light Rule

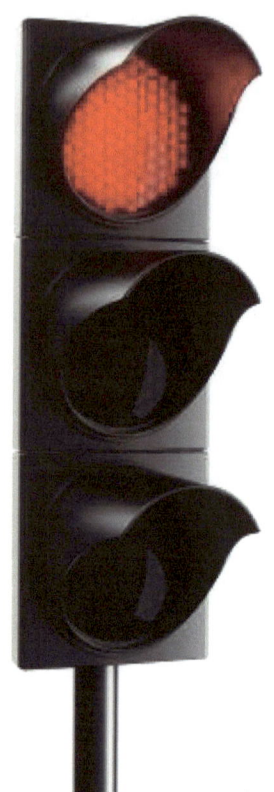

The steps for using the Long Red Light Rule are identical to the Traffic Light Rule, except for Step 7:

7. Circle the first **four** temperatures after Peak Day that are above the coverline: red, red, yellow, green.

You should use the Long Red Light Rule if:
1. You are a beginner.
2. You are confused or your signs of fertility are not matching up.
3. At least one of your 3 elevated temperatures is not 3/10ths of a degree F above the coverline.
4. You have a very serious reason to postpone pregnancy. (In this case, you should wait until 5 of your Post-Peak Day temperatures are above the coverline. You would then circle the first five temperatures: red, red, red, yellow, green.)

**According to the <u>Long Red Light Rule</u>:
You have reached the Luteal Infertile Phase
*on the evening of the cycle day that meets these conditions:***

Since the last day you observed More-Fertile Cervical Fluid,
- **at least four days have passed, AND**
- **<u>four</u> of your temperatures have been above the coverline**

Made in His Image

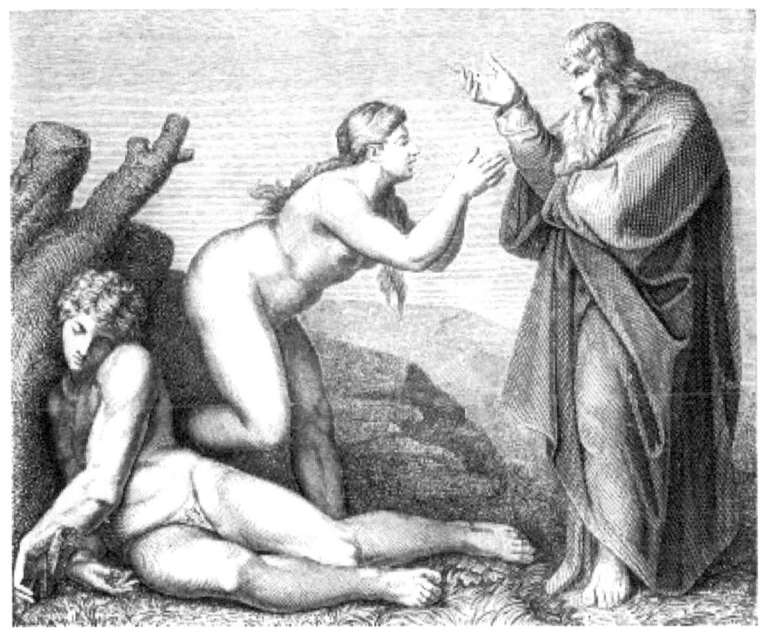

God created man in his image;
in the divine image he created him;
male and female he created them.
~Gen. 1:27 NAB

The Human Body: **Made in His Image**

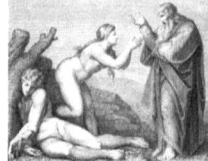

*Discuss the following questions and record your answers. You will need your **Bible** and your copy of **The Human Body: a sign of dignity and a gift.** If you don't know the answer to a question, feel free to skip it.*

I.   Bible Study: Read Genesis 1:26-31

What do you think it means that God created man in His image and likeness?

Do you think it is significant that God created male AND female? Why or why not?

What are the blessings God gave Adam & Eve?

Do you think fruitfulness is a blessing? Why or why not?

Why do you think God commanded Adam & Eve to fill the Earth?

Why do you think God found the creation of humankind "very good"?

II. **Book Study:** Read *The Human Body,* "Introduction," page 1

What document does Fr. Hogan mention that launched the Catholic Church into further developing its teachings on human sexuality, marriage, and family life?

Whose writings especially furthered this development?

What are the names of the two distinct, though inter-related ideas that sum up this development?

What are the main characteristics that define the Theology of the Body, according to Fr. Hogan?

What are the main characteristics of the Theology of the Family?

III. Bible & Book Study: Read Genesis 2:7 and Genesis 2:21-23
Then read *The Human Body,* "Theology of the Body," pages 2-3

Why do man and woman possess "inalienable dignity"?

What is an "incarnate spirit"?

Why do you think John Paul II stated that sexual intercourse is "by no means something purely biological"?

How are human beings different from animals and angels?

What does Fr. Hogan say is the most important principle of the Theology of the Body?

Why do you think Fr. Hogan says the body can be called a "sacrament"?

Why can we never use someone else for our own purposes?

IV.   Bible & Book Study: Read John 15:9-17.
Then read *The Human Body,* "Theology of the Family," pages 3-6

What did Pope Paul VI say is the vocation of every person?

Though they have the same starting position, how are the Theology of the Body & the Theology of the Family different?

What are the five characteristics of God's love, as revealed in Jesus' sacrificial death on the cross?

Why does Fr. Hogan say that the marriage relationship is "the most intimate and intense human relationship of love" aside from one's relationship with God?

What is the defining characteristic of marriage, according to Fr. Hogan?

V.   Discussion

Three Additional Bible & Book Studies:

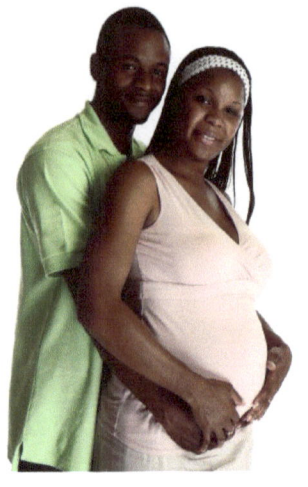

Made to Love as He Loves

We have come to know and to believe in the love God has for us. God is love, and whoever remains in love remains in God and God in him. In this is love brought to perfection among us, that we have confidence on the day of judgment because as he is, so are we in this world... We love because he first loved us.
~ I John 4:16-17 & 19

Made to Give Ourselves

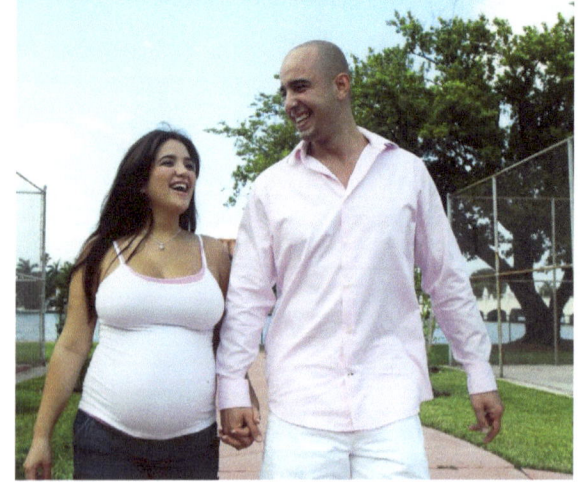

My lover belongs to me and I to him.
~ Song of Songs 6:3

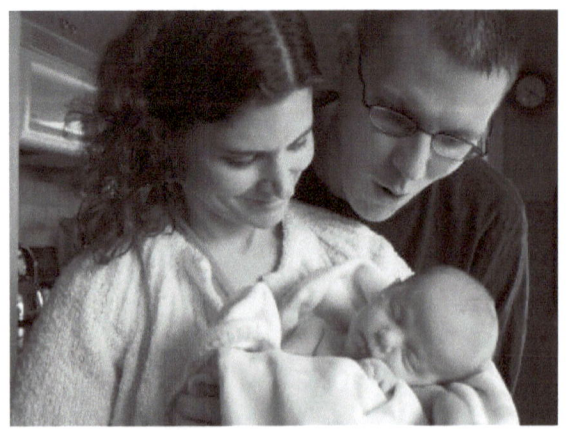

Made to Image God's Love

"Let marriage be held in honor among all, and let the marriage bed be undefiled; for God will judge the immoral and adulterous."
~Hebrews 13:4

The Human Body: **Made to Love as He Loves**

*Discuss the following questions and record your answers. You will need your **Bible** and your copy of **The Human Body: a sign of dignity and a gift.** If you don't know the answer to a question, feel free to skip it.*

I.   **Bible Study:** Read Ephesians 5:28-33

What do you think St. Paul means when he says "husbands should love their wives as their own bodies"?

What are some practical ways a husband might love his wife like his own body?

Why do you think St. Paul wrote that "he who loves his wife loves himself"?

Reflect on the amazing privilege of being a part of Christ's own body (verse 30). In what ways has Christ nourished and cherished you recently?

St. Paul calls marriage a "great mystery" in verse 32. Why?

In what ways is the union of husband and wife like the union of Christ and the Church (cf. verse 32)?

31

Husbands: In what ways can you better love your wife as yourself?

Wives: In what ways can you better respect your husband?

Singles: How can you better show respect and reverence for Christ as your divine spouse?

II.   Book Study: Read *The Human Body,* "Natural Family Planning," pages 6-7

Fr. Hogan identifies one aspect of a person that allows them to love more profoundly than any other physical expression of love. What is it?

When spouses express their love physically in the marriage act, they are a visible image of –whom?

What does the study of Natural Family Planning reveal, according to Fr. Hogan?

Why does the Church encourage individuals to study NFP and human sexuality?

III. Bible & Book Study: Read Psalm 139:13-18 and I Corinthians 7:1-11
Then read *The Human Body,* "Responsible Parenthood," pages 7-12

For each characteristic of divine love, list specific examples of sexual situations where that characteristic is missing.

Choice to give (freely chosen; not coerced):

Informed (based on recognition of the value and dignity of the spouse):

Self-donation (an act of the will to give yourself completely to the other):

Permanent (a binding commitment until death do you part):

Life-Giving (able to transmit human life):

Upon reflection, do you agree that all 5 elements of divine love must be present for sexual intercourse to be a true act of love? Why or why not?

Do you agree that permanence is necessary for a sexual act to be a genuine act of love? Why or why not?

Do you agree that the potential to give life is necessary for genuine love? Why or why not?

What privilege did God give exclusively to human beings?

What is "responsible parenthood' (p.9)?

What is "familial spirituality" (p.10)?

What is the Catholic Church's position on:
  the exclusion of procreation during the marital act?

  the spacing of children using Natural Family Planning?

What does Fr. Hogan report about pastoral experiences with couples who choose to use Natural Family Planning?

Why does Fr. Hogan state that, over the course of time, couples using Natural Family Planning will naturally welcome additional children if they lack serious reasons?

Why do you think Fr. Hogan believes that openness to children is the result of studies of the Theology of the Body, NFP, and the Theology of the Family?

IV.   Discussion

The Human Body: **Made to Give Ourselves**

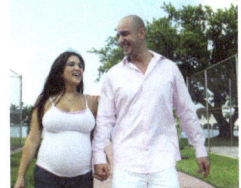

*Discuss the following questions and record your answers. You will need your **Bible** and your copy of **The Human Body: a sign of dignity and a gift.** If you don't know the answer to a question, feel free to skip it.*

I.   **Bible Study:** Read I Corinthians 6:9-20

What is your reaction to how seriously St. Paul regards the sins listed in verses 9 & 10? Does the inclusion in this list of any of these sins surprise you? Why or why not?

What does it mean to be washed?   Sanctified?   Justified?

St. Paul quotes a very modern-sounding maxim reflecting moral relativism: "Everything is lawful for me." How does he refute the belief that sexual behavior is a moral "gray zone"?

What does St. Paul mean when he says that the body is for the Lord (verse 13)?

What do you think he means when he says the Lord is for the body?

What is the significance of the Resurrection when discussing sexual morality (verse 14)?

What does it mean to sin against your own body (verse 18)?

In what ways can you better glorify God with your body, as St. Paul exhorts in verse 20?

II. **Book Study:** Read *The Human Body,* "Sins," pages 13-14

What does Fr. Hogan identify as the foundation of the Catholic Church's teaching on the dignity of the human person and the vocation of marriage?

What causes human beings to struggle so much with living according to our own dignity?

What are the effects of original sin on our bodies?

What aspect of our person has been particularly damaged by original sin?

What happens when we act on our sexual desires without the temperance of our wills and minds? What do we fail to do?

III. Book Study: Read *The Human Body,* "Sins," pages 14-27, starting with the section called "Lust" and ending with the "Conclusion." For each sin discussed in this portion of the booklet, record if these characteristic(s) of divine love are *present* in this action (yes, no, sometimes, ?, n/a).

Sinful Action	Choice (an action you have freely chosen; not coerced)	Informed (done with recognition of the value & dignity of the other)	Self-Gift (done following an act of the will to give yourself completely to the other)	Permanence (done following a binding commitment to remain with the other until death)	Life-Giving (action that is able to transmit human life)
Lust					
Pornography					
Intimate Touching					
Masturbation					
Extramarital Sexual Activity					
Divorce & Remarriage					
Contraception & Sterilization					
Artificial Reproductive Techniques					
Abortion					
Homosexual Activity					

IV. **Reflection & Prayer:** Reflect on which of these sins (whether your personal sin or the sins of others) have had the most damaging effects throughout your life. Ask for God's help to overcome the damaging effects of original sin today and in the future. Ask for His grace to authentically love all those with whom you come in contact. Thank the Lord for the ways He has helped you to avoid sin, the ways He has already healed you, and how He has helped you to grow in self-mastery.

V. **Book Study:** Read *The Human Body,* "Formation of Conscience (Veritatis Splendor)," pages 27-31.

What is a conscience?

What is the distinction between the conscience *evaluating* what is good and evil and the conscience *determining* if an act is good or evil?

What are some practical consequences of the popular belief that one's conscience is the source of truth—for the individual *and* for society?

Do you think Fr. Hogan is correct in his assessment that if each person were to determine the moral law for himself, the result would be dictatorship or rule by mob? Why or why not?

What did John Paul II mean when he wrote "conscience has rights because it has duties"?

What sources of truth help to inform one's conscience?

What do you think a person should do if he discovers that one of his actions is immoral that he thought was moral? Can you think of examples in your own life, whether currently or in the past?

What do you think a person should do if he discovers that an action is considered immoral, yet he does not understand or agree? Can you think of examples in your own life, whether currently or in the past?

VI. Discussion

The Human Body: **Made to Image God's Love**

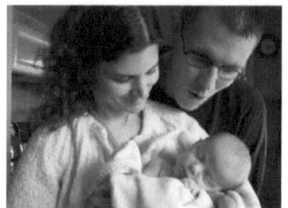

*Discuss the following questions and record your answers. You will need your **Bible** and your copy of **The Human Body: a sign of dignity and a gift.** If you don't know the answer to a question, feel free to skip it.*

I.   Bible Study: Read John 2: 1-11

Why do you think Mary asked Jesus to help the bridal couple when the wine ran out?

Why do you think Jesus performed the miracle of changing water into wine, even after He said that His "hour" had not yet come?

What are some possible meanings of the good wine?

Jesus' first miracle occurred at a wedding feast, a sign of His blessing upon all marriages. If you are married, how have you experienced God's blessing upon your marriage?

Mary told the servants to "do whatever he tells you" in verse 5. Has Jesus impressed anything on you throughout the study of Scripture and/or this book study that you believe He wants you to do?

II. **Book Study:** Read *The Human Body,* "Marriage as a Sacrament," pages 32-35

How is marriage a sign of how God loves us?

How is marriage an image of the Trinity?

How is marriage a sign of how Christ loves the Church?

What is the gift God gives that enables us to love as He loves?

What is "sacramental" about marriage (whether yours, or marriages in general)?

What is the sign of the sacrament of marriage?

How does a family (husband, wife and children) imitate the Trinity?

How can you better image God's love to others in your life?

If married, how can your marriage better image God's love to those around you?

III. Reflection and Prayer of Thanksgiving

The wine which Jesus made was "good." Reflect on the "good wine" Our Lord has made from the "empty jars" and plain "water" of your life. Recall the many times He has taken your emptiness and ordinariness and transformed them into abundance and joy. Consider God's many blessings and the graces He has given you, and spend some time in prayer thanking Him.

IV. Discussion

The Natural Fertility Support Program...

- Promotes healthy habits that naturally encourage healthy fertility

- The Principles of the Natural Fertility Support Program are:
  - Eat a healthy diet and drink plenty of clean water.
  - Exercise regularly, but moderately.
  - Plan your life to achieve a balance of worship, work, rest, sleep, and recreation.

- The Natural Fertility Support program is taught throughout the series:
  - This Session: overview of the program
  - 2nd Session: Super Foods for Super Fertility (nutrition & fertility)
  - 3rd Session: Exercising Your Way to Better Health (exercise & fertility)
  - Fertility Counseling Appointments: The GIFTs of Life & Love goal-setting process

Nurturing the GIFTs of Life & Love

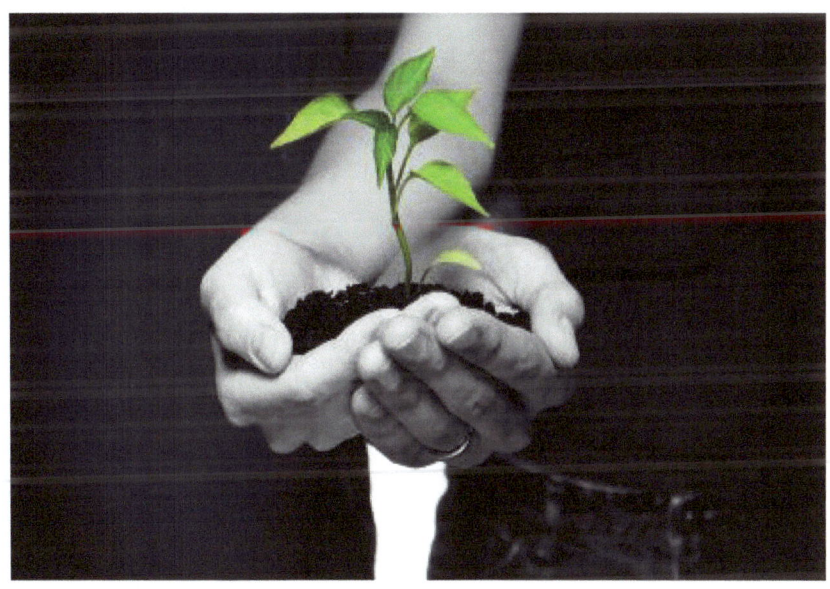

First we make our habits, then our habits make us.
~Charles C. Noble

Nurturing the GIFTs of Life & Love

- Your fertility in part reflects your lifestyle

- Your lifestyle is set by your habits

- We all have healthy habits that we want to maintain and unhealthy habits we would like to change

- Planning our habits and writing them down helps us to make progress toward the specific changes we would like to make

- Having someone to keep us accountable also helps us to change

- Change requires self-discipline/self-control

- Self-control is a fruit of the spirit (Gal. 5:22)

- Jesus has promised that if we ask, we shall receive (Matt. 7:7); we need to ask Him for divine help and the gift of self-control

- By growing closer to God, we will be better equipped to accept all circumstances

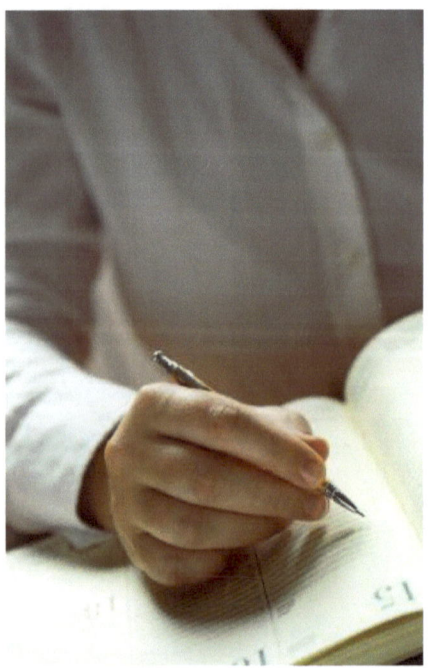

Objective: **To Help You Become a Better GIFT, so you can give yourself in love**

G God First

- Spiritual Growth: Growth in holiness is the foundation, the means, and the ultimate goal of the Fertility Matters™ Method
- Growth in Chastity: Whether married or not, everyone needs to continue to grow in chastity, especially with the increasing temptations in the culture around us. You will be encouraged to view this virtue as the source of joy and peace that it truly is.

I Me, myself and I next

- Improved Overall Health: You will set your own practical, achievable self-care goals that have demonstrated effectiveness in improving health, including fertility. The Fertility Matters™ Method is evidence-based.
- Increased Peace and Joy in one's Daily Life: The Fertility Matters™ Method includes caring for yourself, reducing stress and cultivating relationships and activities that bring joy into your life.

F Family Next

- Stronger Marriages: If you are married, living in harmony with your fertility and resisting the world's "quick fixes" can be very trying on a marriage—whether your intention is to conceive or to postpone pregnancy. This program leads you to keep making your marriage a priority and to plan your family through only marriage-strengthening means.
- Attached Families: What means more to children than the love & time of their parents?
- A Stable Financial Foundation & Sufficient Possessions: You must provide for yourself and your family—and not just with finances—providing good meals, clean clothes, and loving care of your home are ways you provide, too!

T Lastly, **The World** needs YOU!

- Spread the Gospel of Life and Love: After covering the most important priorities first, the time remaining is for helping to spread the gospel of life and practice the works of mercy!

The Fertility Matters™ Method...

- Includes the **Nurturing the GIFTs of Life & Love** Goal-Setting Process to inspire you and give you the skills to make the changes that move you closer to becoming the type of person that God wants you to be and the person that you want to become

- Nurturing the GIFTs of Life & Love is a **goal setting process** which covers all six main areas of a person's life:
    - **Spiritual**
    - **Personal**
    - **Marital** (for married)
    - **Parenting** (for parents)
    - **Vocational** & **Financial**
    - **Relationships & Needs Outside of Yourself and Your Family**: Extended Family, Neighborhood, Church Family, Friendships, Missions, Apostolates, Ministries, Volunteering, Serving the Poor, etc.

- Your fertility advisor provides a built-in accountability partner to help you work toward your goals!

Steps

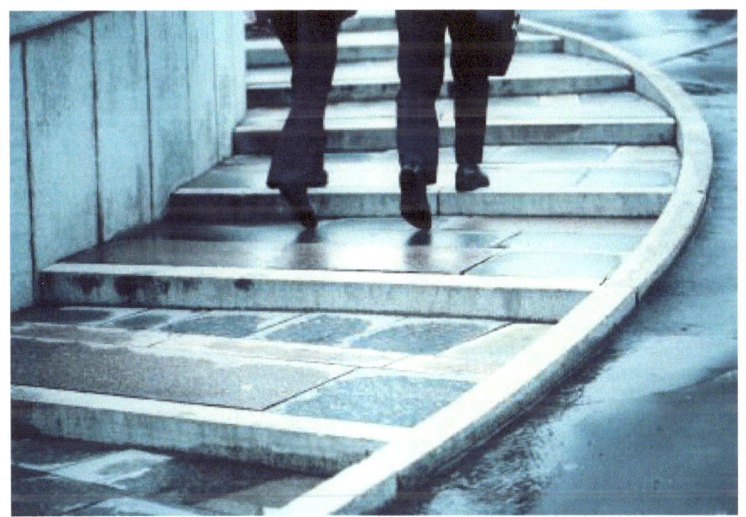

*The vision must be followed by the venture.
It is not enough to stare up the steps—
we must step up the stairs.
~Vance Havner, American Baptist preacher*

Steps in the Fertility Matters™ Method During the Course

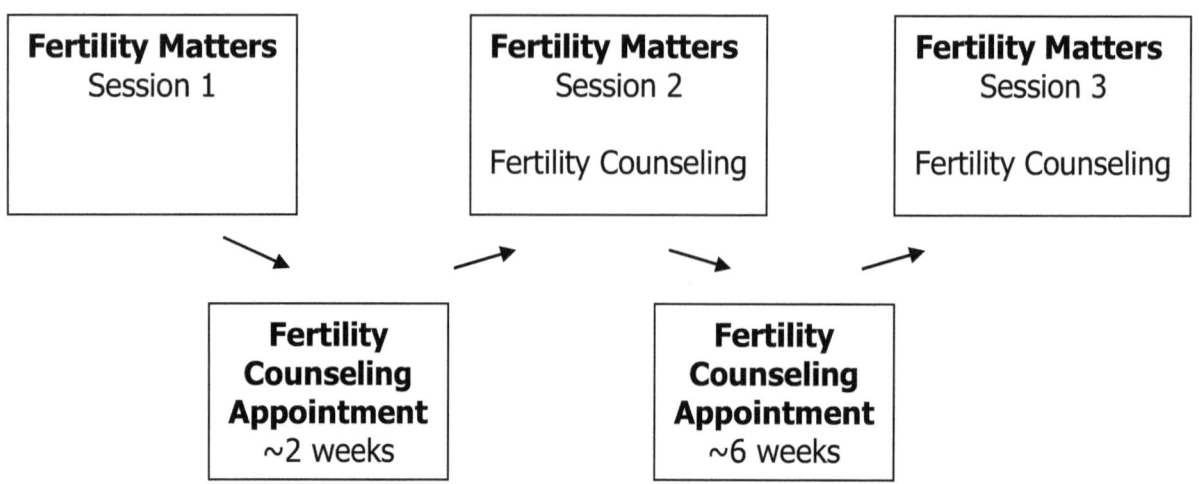

| Fertility Matters Session 1 | Fertility Matters Session 2 — Fertility Counseling | Fertility Matters Session 3 — Fertility Counseling |

Fertility Counseling Appointment ~2 weeks

Fertility Counseling Appointment ~6 weeks

Following the Course

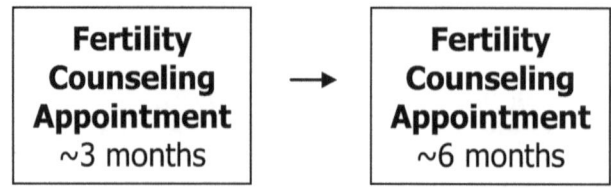

Fertility Counseling Appointment ~3 months → **Fertility Counseling Appointment** ~6 months

Our GIFT Goals

G <u>G</u>od First

I Me, myself and <u>I</u> next

F <u>F</u>amily Next
- *Marriage:*

- *Family:*

- *Financial Foundation & Other Provision:*

T Lastly, **The World** needs YOU!
Spreading the Gospel of Life and Love:

Remember to write "SMART" Goals:

S=Specific
M=Measurable
A=Agreed Upon
R=Realistic
T=Timely

www.ingramcontent.com/pod-product-compliance
Lightning Source LLC
Chambersburg PA
CBHW041512280526
45792CB00004B/1227